Mitochondrial Dynamics

Bridging The Gap Between Health And Dysfunction

Raphael Jason

Table of Contents

Introduction (Key ideas)
Chapter One
1.1 Overview of Mitochondrial Dynamics
1.2 Significance in Cellular Function.
"Fundamentals of Fusion and Fission"
Chapter Two
2.1 Mitochondrial Fusion: Creating Cellular Networks.
2.2 Mitochondrial Fission: Division for Cellular Health Balancing Act in Cellular Health.
Chapter Three
3.1 Equilibrium Between Fusion and Fission
3.2 Role in Energy Production and Cellular Resilience Molecular Mechanisms Governing Dynamics.
Chapter Four
4.1 Key Proteins and Regulators
4.2 Cellular Signaling and Apoptosis Regulation Impact of Dysfunction on Mitochondrial Dynamics.
Chapter Five
5.1 Fragmentation and Elongation: Consequences of Imbalance.

5.2 Link to Various Pathologies: Neurodegenerative Disorders, Metabolic Syndromes, Cardiovascular Diseases Bridging the Gap: Understanding the Molecular Basis.

Chapter Six

6.1 Investigating Molecular Mechanisms.

6.2 Technological Advances in Studying Mitochondrial Dynamics Therapeutic Approaches.

Chapter Seven

7.1 Small Molecule Interventions.

7.2 CRISPR-based Strategies for Modulation Future Perspectives.

Chapter Eight

8.1 Emerging Research Avenues

8.2 Potential Implications for Disease Treatment Conclusion

Chapter Nine

9.1 Summarizing the Key Findings

9.2 Looking Ahead: Implications for Cellular and Medical Research

Conclusion

General Assessment Questions

Introduction

(Key ideas)

Maintaining optimal mitochondrial activity is critical for energy production and other fundamental cellular functions, and it is largely dependent on mitochondrial dynamics. This mechanism, which is essential for the best possible function in signal transduction and metabolism, is the shifting process of fission, fusion, mitophagy, and transport. Numerous illnesses, such as cancer, metabolic, cardiovascular, and neurological diseases, are linked to imbalanced mitochondrial dynamics. This review aims to clarify the role of mitochondrial dynamics in bridging the gap between health and dysfunction by examining the machinery involved in mitochondrial dynamics and their dysfunction in disease.

As the primary producers of adenosine triphosphate (ATP), the chemical energy source that cells use, mitochondria are referred to as the powerhouses of the cell. Apart from generating energy, mitochondria are engaged in various additional functions like controlling cellular demise, maintaining calcium balance, and generating reactive oxygen species (ROS).

To keep the number of mitochondria in the cell healthy, fission, fusion, transport, and destruction are all aspects of mitochondrial dynamics. Mitochondria can adjust to fluctuating energy requirements, heal damage, and eliminate unhealthy mitochondria through several activities.

Numerous disorders can result from imbalances in the dynamics of the mitochondria. For instance, too much fission can result in the creation of broken, malfunctioning mitochondria, which are linked to neurological conditions like Parkinson's and Alzheimer's disease. On the other hand, poor fusion is linked to illnesses such as dominant optic atrophy and Charcot-Marie-Tooth disease because it can result in the buildup of damaged mitochondrial DNA.

Research is being done to better understand the mechanisms that control mitochondrial dynamics and how they affect disease. Mitochondrial dynamics is a viable target for the development of novel therapeutics for various diseases, as it bridges the gap between health and dysfunction.

You can use this book as a tool to support your personal development and growth. The benefits will be increased by your commitment to actively participating in the activities and critically evaluating your development. "Mitochondrial dynamics: Bridging the gap between health and dysfunction" is a fun topic to explore, and it might result in a beneficial and long-lasting improvement in your life.

Feel free to assess your understanding and application of the concepts in the book here. Evaluate your overall progression and recommend areas that still require improvement.

Chapter One

1.1 Overview of Mitochondrial Dynamics

The ongoing processes of fission, fusion, mitophagy, and transport are referred to as "mitochondrial dynamics," and they are essential for preserving optimal mitochondrial function and directing different cellular processes. Because of their dynamic nature, mitochondria are able to adapt to various stressors and metabolic requirements within a cell, demonstrating their plasticity. Disrupted mitochondrial function can result from imbalances in mitochondrial dynamics, which can lead to aberrant cellular destiny and a variety of illnesses, such as malignancies, metabolic diseases, cardiovascular diseases, and neurodegenerative disorders.

- Mitochondrial Dynamics Mechanisms.

Large GTPases from the Dynamin family control the coordinated cycles of fission and fusion that are part of mitochondrial dynamics. While two mitochondria can fuse together to form a single organelle, one mitochondrion can divide into two daughter mitochondria in a process known as mitochondrial fission.

- Function in Illness and Health.

Ensuring mitochondrial function and meeting cellular demands depend on maintaining appropriate mitochondrial dynamics. A number of clinical disorders have been linked to imbalanced mitochondrial dynamics, underscoring the importance of these dynamic transitions for cellular health.

- Possible Modulation Targets.

Determining how mitochondrial form meets function and learning more about the underlying causes of disorders linked to morphological abnormalities depend on an understanding of the molecular mechanisms governing mitochondrial dynamics. A new avenue for the development of more accurate techniques for the targeted regulation of mitochondrial function is to target the modification of mitochondrial dynamics.

- Implications for Treating Illnesses

It has been demonstrated that improving mitochondrial fitness through control of mitochondrial dynamics lowers the risk of illness and improves cellular health in general. Consequently, it is crucial to conduct research to determine whether mitochondrial dynamics might be used as a target for the prevention and treatment of age-related diseases.

In conclusion, abnormalities in this process can result in a variety of disorders. Mitochondrial dynamics are crucial for preserving good mitochondrial function. In the context of mitochondrial-related disorders, comprehending the molecular mechanisms and possible targets for modifying mitochondrial dynamics is crucial for formulating methods to close the gap between health and dysfunction.

1.2 Significance in Cellular Function.

"Fundamentals of Fusion and Fission"

The processes of fusion and fission in the mitochondria are essential for preserving the integrity and functionality of cells. Mitochondria may adjust to changing cellular needs and pressures thanks to this ongoing process, which guarantees optimal function and quality control.

Fission vs Fusion

Fission, which is controlled by DRP1 and FIS1, is the division of a mitochondrion into two daughter mitochondria, whereas mitotic fusion, which is the joining of two mitochondria, is aided by big GTPases such MFN1, MFN2, and OPA1. For cellular homeostasis and function, these activities regulate the shape, distribution, and interchange of material within the mitochondria[5].

Importance for Cellular Activity

Because mitochondrial fusion and fission are dynamic processes, they can quickly respond to changes in metabolic demands and cellular stress, which helps to maintain a healthy population of mitochondria. A number of illnesses, including neurodegenerative diseases, have been related to imbalances in fusion and fission, underscoring the vital role that mitochondrial dynamics play in maintaining cellular health.

Consequences for Dysfunction and Health
Maintaining mitochondrial integrity, function, and quality control requires proper dynamics within the mitochondria. Dysfunctional dynamics can eventually contribute to the pathophysiology of disease by reducing mitochondrial fitness, making cells more susceptible to apoptosis, and impairing cellular metabolism.

To sum up, the basic mechanisms of mitochondrial fusion and fission are what distinguish healthy cells from unhealthy ones. It is imperative to comprehend the molecular mechanisms and relevance of these dynamic events in order to clarify their role in the development of diseases and to devise focused therapies aimed at preserving normal mitochondrial function.

Chapter Two

2.1 Mitochondrial Fusion: Creating Cellular Networks.

In order to dilute malfunctioning proteins and altered mtDNA, a process known as mitochondrial fusion entails combining mitochondrial proteins, mtDNA, and other matrix elements. For signal transduction and metabolism to operate as best they can, fission, fusion, mitophagy, and transport must all change. This process is known as mitochondrial dynamics. Disruption of mitochondrial function due to an imbalance in mitochondrial dynamics can result in various diseases such as malignancies, metabolic disorders, neurological disorders, and cardiovascular diseases, as well as incorrect cellular fate. Neurodegenerative illnesses can result from an imbalance of mitochondrial dynamics caused by dysfunction in the main fission and fusion machinery components, such as dynamin-related protein 1 (DRP1), mitofusins 1 and 2 (MFN1, MFN2), and optic atrophy protein 1 (OPA1). More prevalent illnesses also have altered mitochondrial dynamics. Because of the fundamental roles that mitochondria play in human physiology, "mitochondrial dysfunction" has been linked to a broad spectrum of illnesses that affect every facet of medicine.

2.2 Mitochondrial Fission: Division for Cellular Health Balancing Act in Cellular Health.

The process by which a mitochondrion splits into two mitochondria is known as mitochondrial fission, and it is crucial for preserving the number and appropriate distribution of mitochondria within the cell. When there is an imbalance with mitochondrial fusion, this process, which is essential for mitochondrial division and quality control, is linked to a number of illnesses, including cancer, neurological, and cardiovascular diseases. Contrarily, mitochondrial fusion enables the transfer of gene products between mitochondria for optimal performance, particularly in the presence of environmental and metabolic stress. Cellular homeostasis depends on the proper balance between fusion and fission; when this equilibrium is upset, many diseases can arise as a result of changes to the number, structure, and functionality of mitochondria.

Therefore, maintaining cellular health and preventing disease require a precise balance between mitochondrial fusion and fission.

Chapter Three

3.1 Equilibrium Between Fusion and Fission

Dynamic organelles, mitochondria go through processes called fusion and fission that are essential for preserving cellular homeostasis and optimum function. For mitochondrial morphology and function, fusion and fission must be balanced; an imbalance can result in a number of illnesses, such as cancer, metabolic diseases, and neurodegenerative disorders. A number of age-related disorders are linked to mitochondrial dysfunction, which is brought on by flaws in the dynamics of the mitochondria. In order to remove damaged mitochondrial components and eliminate compromised or malfunctioning mitochondria to stop additional cellular damage, the balance between fusion and fission is essential.

To close the gap between mitochondrial dynamics in health and dysfunction, it is crucial to comprehend the molecular mechanisms and biological roles of mitochondrial fusion and fission.

3.2 Role in Energy Production and Cellular Resilience Molecular Mechanisms Governing Dynamics.

Cellular resilience and energy generation are significantly influenced by mitochondria. They are the main organelles that control how much energy the cell produces and how long it can withstand stress. For signal transmission and metabolism to perform as best they can, mitochondrial dynamics—which encompass the processes of fusion, fission, mitophagy, and transport—are essential. Disruption of mitochondrial function due to an imbalance in mitochondrial dynamics can result in aberrant cellular destiny and a variety of illnesses, such as malignancies, metabolic diseases, cardiovascular diseases, and neurodegenerative disorders. The preservation of mitochondrial integrity and homeostasis depends on the biological roles and molecular processes of mitochondrial fusion and fission. While fission is essential for mitochondrial division and quality control, mitochondrial fusion permits the transfer of gene products between mitochondria for optimal functioning, particularly under metabolic and environmental stress. Numerous illnesses, including cancer, neurological, and cardiovascular disorders, are linked to the equilibrium between these two processes. Disorders of mitochondrial dynamics are a class of mitochondrial diseases caused by defects in fission and fusion-related mitochondrial proteins caused by pathogenic variations in the genes encoding these proteins. This disturbs the equilibrium between fission and fusion. Thus, bridging the gap between health and dysfunction in mitochondrial dynamics requires an understanding of the molecular mechanisms and biological roles of mitochondrial fusion and fission.

Chapter Four

4.1 Key Proteins and Regulators

Key Proteins and Controllers in Mitochondrial Functions.

The processes of fission, fusion, mitophagy, and transport are known as mitochondrial dynamics, and they are essential for metabolism and signal transduction to operate at their best. Disruption of mitochondrial function due to imbalanced dynamics in the mitochondria can result in aberrant cellular destiny and various diseases such as malignancies, metabolic diseases, cardiovascular diseases, and neurodegenerative disorders. The essential proteins and regulators in mitochondrial dynamics and their function in bridging the gap between health and dysfunction will be covered in this article.

- Proteins Involved in Mitotic Fusion.

A number of proteins control mitochondrial fusion, including:

1. Mitofusins 1 and 2 (MFN1 and MFN2): These proteins are vital for preserving the healthy

function of mitochondria and are involved in the fusion process.

2. Optimin-alpha (OPA1): This protein is essential for preserving the equilibrium between mitochondrial division and fusion and is also involved in the fusion process

- Fission Proteins in Mitochondria

A number of proteins control mitochondrial fission, including:

1. Dynamin-related protein 1 (DRP1): DRP1 is critical for preserving the ideal balance between mitochondrial division and fusion and is involved in the fission process.

2. Fission protein 1 (FIS1): FIS1 is an additional fission-related protein that has been linked to mitochondrial malfunction and fragmentation.

- Modifications Made After Translation.

The function of mitochondrial dynamics proteins is significantly regulated by post-translational modifications, or PTMs. Among these changes include ubiquitination, glycosylation, and phosphorylation. Comprehending the interaction between these PTMs and the molecular and cellular mechanisms that underpin mitochondrial dynamics provides significant understanding of the pathogenesis of various illnesses, including neurodegenerative diseases.

- The Dynamics of Mitochondria in Disease

Numerous illnesses, including malignancies, metabolic disorders, cardiovascular disorders, and neurological diseases have been linked to dysregulation of mitochondrial dynamics. It is feasible to create more precise techniques for targeted regulation of mitochondrial function by focusing on the modulation of mitochondrial dynamics, which lowers the risk of disease and improves the quality of life for those who are affected.

In conclusion, designing tailored therapeutic techniques aiming at restoring or maintaining correct mitochondrial dynamics requires an understanding of the key proteins and regulators in mitochondrial dynamics as well as their involvement in health and sickness. This information may offer a fresh strategy for treating crippling illnesses and enhancing the quality of life for those with mitochondrial dysfunction.

4.2 Cellular Signaling and Apoptosis Regulation Impact of Dysfunction on Mitochondrial Dynamics.

Regulation of Apoptosis and Cellular Signaling

The control of cellular signaling and apoptosis, a type of predetermined cell death, is largely dependent on mitochondria. Abnormal cellular destiny and various diseases, such as malignancies, metabolic diseases, cardiovascular diseases, and neurodegenerative disorders, can result from dysfunction in mitochondrial dynamics.

Apoptosis and Mitochondrial Dynamics

Through a number of pathways, mitochondria contribute to apoptotic cell death.

1. Pro-apoptotic molecule release: Chromosome condensation and fragmentation are caused by mitochondria, which also release pro-apoptotic chemicals and activate caspases.

2. Intrinsic and extrinsic mechanisms for apoptosis: Apoptosis can be initiated by either intrinsic or

extrinsic pathway. The intrinsic route causes the pro-apoptotic BCL-2 family proteins Bax/Bak to become active. This leads to the creation of pores in the outer mitochondrial membrane (OMM) and the release of cytochrome c (Cyt C) into the cytoplasm, which triggers caspases and starts the apoptotic process.

3. Mitochondrial outer membrane permeabilization: After being released into the cytoplasm, some proteins, including cytochrome c, are sequestered by mitochondria and subsequently activate caspases directly. This causes nuclear condensation and blebbing of the plasma membrane, two morphological changes that are typical of apoptotic cell death

Effect of Dysfunction on Dynamics of Mitochondria.

A variety of cellular functions are impacted by mitochondrial malfunction, which is closely linked to abnormal mitochondrial dynamics. These processes include:

- Cell cycle regulation - Mitochondrial transport and biogenesis - Cell proliferation and differentiation

The processes of energy metabolism, ROS generation, Ca2+ signaling, mtDNA maintenance, and autophagic (mitophagous) mitochondrial quality control

Pro- and anti-apoptotic proteins, including Bcl-2, Bcl-XL, Bcl-W, and MCL1, can become unbalanced due to dysfunction in mitochondrial dynamics. These proteins are essential for controlling programmed cell death. An imbalance may cause apoptosis to be triggered, which would then cause illness and malfunctioning cells.

Disease and Mitochondrial Dynamics

Numerous pathological disorders have been linked to mitochondrial dynamics, including:

Hypoxia, medication therapies, neurological conditions, metabolic illnesses, cardiovascular conditions, and cancers.

Gaining knowledge of the mechanisms behind mitochondrial dynamics and how they affect cellular signaling and the regulation of apoptosis can be extremely helpful in the development of novel therapeutic approaches for the treatment of disorders linked to mitochondrial malfunction.

Regulation of Apoptosis and Cellular Signaling

The control of cellular signaling and apoptosis, a type of predetermined cell death, is largely dependent on mitochondria. Abnormal cellular destiny and various diseases, such as malignancies, metabolic diseases, cardiovascular diseases, and neurodegenerative disorders, can result from dysfunction in mitochondrial dynamics.

Chapter Five

5.1 Fragmentation and Elongation: Consequences of Imbalance.

Disintegration and Extension: Effects of Disproportionality in Mitochondrial Motion

The processes of fission, fusion, mitophagy, and transport—all essential for optimal performance in signal transduction and metabolism—are referred to as mitochondrial dynamics . Disruption of mitochondrial function due to an imbalance in mitochondrial dynamics can result in aberrant cellular destiny and a variety of illnesses, such as malignancies, metabolic diseases, cardiovascular diseases, and neurodegenerative disorders. The effects of mitochondrial dynamics' fragmentation and elongation on both health and dysfunction will be covered in this article.

- Disintegration of Mitochondria.

Fission, or excessive division of the mitochondria, is linked to functional abnormalities and has been linked to a number of human illnesses, including cancer and neurological diseases[2]. Unbalanced fusion and fission processes cause mitochondrial malfunction, which in turn causes mtDNA depletion, ROS generation, mitochondrial fragmentation, and loss of oxidative phosphorylation (OXPHOS). For instance, an imbalance in mitochondrial dynamics is observed in Alzheimer's disease, where aberrantly fragmented mitochondria are discovered as a result of increased expression of fission factors and decreased production of fusion proteins.

- Extension of the Mitochondrion

However, the suppression of fission can also result in mitochondrial elongation. It has been observed that inflammatory responses are dependent on the morphology of the mitochondria. An NFκB-dependent inflammatory response is associated with mitochondrial fragmentation caused by inhibition of fusion, while an NFκB-dependent inflammatory response is activated by mitochondrial elongation caused by inhibition of fission.

- Imbalanced Mitochondrial Dynamics' Consequences

Inflammation can be induced by mtDNA mislocation, which is facilitated by imbalances in mitochondrial dynamics and is dependent on the shape of the mitochondria. For example, mitochondrial elongation can activate the type I IFN response and NFκB-dependent pathways, whereas mitochondrial fragmentation can cause inflammation. In addition to other chronic inflammation-related illnesses and disorders associated with mitochondrial malfunction, these inflammatory responses may play a role in the development of atrophy and its complications.

- Putting Mitochondrial Dynamics in Focus.

Different methods for modifying mitochondrial morphology can produce various inflammatory patterns. More exact methods for the targeted regulation of mitochondrial activity can be developed by comprehending the molecular mechanisms of mitochondrial dynamics and their effects on health and disease. This may result in the development of novel therapeutic strategies for the treatment of conditions marked by mitochondrial malfunction and chronic inflammation.

In conclusion, aberrant dynamics causing mitochondria to fragment and elongate can have serious effects on both health and dysfunction. Comprehending the underlying principles of these processes and their effects on cellular function can aid in the creation of innovative therapeutic approaches for a range of ailments. To fully comprehend the complexities of mitochondrial dynamics and their function in preserving cellular health, more investigation is required.

5.2 Link to Various Pathologies: Neurodegenerative Disorders, Metabolic Syndromes, Cardiovascular Diseases Bridging the Gap: Understanding the Molecular Basis.

Connection to a Range of Pathologies: Metabolic Syndromes, Cardiovascular Diseases, Neurodegenerative Disorders

Maintaining optimal mitochondrial activity is critical for energy production and other critical cellular functions, and it is largely dependent on mitochondrial dynamics. Disturbances in the dynamics of the mitochondria can impair the function of the mitochondria, resulting in aberrant cellular destiny and a variety of illnesses, such as malignancies, metabolic diseases, neurological disorders, and cardiovascular diseases. The relationship between mitochondrial dynamics and several pathologies will be covered in this section, with an emphasis on metabolic syndromes, cardiovascular diseases, and neurodegenerative disorders.

- Degenerative Conditions.

The onset and course of neurodegenerative disorders, including Alzheimer's disease (AD), are linked to mitochondrial dynamics. Due to an imbalance in mitochondrial dynamics caused by increased expression of fission factors and decreased expression of fusion proteins, AD is associated with aberrantly fragmented mitochondria. The development of amyloid-beta plaques and the ensuing neurodegeneration seen in AD are both facilitated by this imbalance.

- Syndromes of Metabolism.

Diabetes and obesity are two metabolic disorders whose pathogenesis is linked to mitochondrial dysfunction. Neuropathies such as Charcot-Marie-Tooth disease, where mitochondrial fusion and transport are compromised, or dominant optic atrophy, where there is a decrease in mitochondrial fusion, can be brought on by changes in mitochondrial dynamics. Primary mitochondrial illnesses resulting in dysfunctional mitochondria lead to the generation of reactive oxygen species, which in turn affects the mitochondria's function and dynamics. This creates a vicious cycle that persists and intensifies the diseased phenotype.

- Cardiovascular Conditions.

Cardiovascular disorders can arise as a result of aberrations in mitochondrial dynamics, which are crucial for preserving cardiovascular health. For instance, excessive mitochondrial division, or fission, has been linked to a number of human disorders, including cardiovascular conditions. Numerous cardiovascular diseases have been linked to mitochondrial dysfunction, and sustaining cardiovascular health depends on the appropriate clearance of malfunctioning mitochondria.

In summary, the genesis and progression of numerous illnesses, such as metabolic syndromes, cardiovascular diseases, and neurodegenerative disorders, are significantly influenced by mitochondrial dynamics. Gaining insight into the molecular underpinnings of mitochondrial dynamics and how they affect health and illness might aid in the development of more focused tactics for the targeted regulation of mitochondrial activity, which may result in the creation of novel therapeutic methods for various conditions.

Chapter Six

6.1 Investigating Molecular Mechanisms.

The active organelles known as mitochondria are essential to preserving cellular activity. For mitochondria to perform as best they can, a variety of mechanisms including fission, fusion, mitophagy, and transport are part of the mitochondrial dynamics. Disruptive mitochondria can result from imbalances in mitochondrial dynamics, and these can be linked to a variety of illnesses, such as cancer, metabolic diseases, cardiovascular diseases, and neurodegenerative disorders.

Studies have demonstrated the involvement of defective mitochondria in the etiology of cardiovascular aging and heart disease. Through control of morphology, content exchange, mitochondrial heredity, maintenance of mitochondrial DNA, and autophagy's elimination of damaged mitochondria, mitochondrial dynamics—including fusion, fission, and motility—are crucial for preserving mitochondrial homeostasis.

Mitophagy is a crucial step in maintaining the quality of mitochondria by destroying defective mitochondria in a targeted manner. Serious repercussions from damaged or dysfunctional mitochondria can include increased oxidative stress and cell death. Numerous disorders, including cardiovascular conditions including myocardial infarction, cardiomyopathy, and heart failure, are directly linked to the etiology of mitophagy.

All things considered, learning more about the molecular mechanisms behind mitochondrial dynamics is essential to comprehending the link between health and dysfunction. It may shed light on how to create exact plans for the focused control of mitochondrial activity, which could have consequences for the management of a number of illnesses.

6.2 Technological Advances in Studying Mitochondrial Dynamics Therapeutic Approaches.

The shifting processes of fission, fusion, mitophagy, and transport are referred to as mitochondrial dynamics. These processes are essential for the best possible performance in signal transduction and metabolism. A variety of illnesses that are commonly characterized by decreased mitochondrial function and increased cell death are linked to imbalanced mitochondrial dynamics. There is growing evidence that changes in mitochondrial dynamics play a role in multiple facets of carcinogenesis and the advancement of cancer.

Therefore, one possible therapeutic strategy for the treatment of cancer would be to target the regulator of mitochondrial dynamics. In a number of illness models, improving mitochondrial fusion and division through genetic or small chemical manipulation has improved function. A thorough grasp of mitochondrial dynamics will help researchers create more accurate plans for focused modulation of mitochondrial function.

Chapter Seven

7.1 Small Molecule Interventions.

Maintaining optimal mitochondrial activity is critical for energy production and other fundamental cellular functions, and it is largely dependent on mitochondrial dynamics. Studies have been conducted on small-molecule interventions as a possible means of controlling mitochondrial dynamics and bridging the gap between normal and pathological conditions. For instance, a 2023 study that was published in Nature Chemical Biology described the use of S89, a small chemical agonist, to precisely stimulate mitochondrial fusion by targeting endogenous MFN1, hence correcting dysfunction-related cellular and mitochondrial defects.

The apparatus involved in mitochondrial dynamics and their malfunction in disease were the subject of another study published in FEBS Letters. These results point to the potential benefit of small-molecule therapies focusing on mitochondrial dynamics in treating mitochondrial malfunction and related health issues.

Furthermore, studies on small-molecule treatments that target mitochondrial dysfunction in the aging and degeneration of the intervertebral disc are being conducted. A review paper addressing the pathophysiology of mitochondrial failure in intervertebral disc aging and degeneration was published in the NCBI in 2021. It also highlighted the possible significance of small molecules in addressing this dysfunction.

According to the article, a potential treatment approach for intervertebral disc degeneration could use small-molecule therapies that target mitochondrial dysfunction. All things considered, these results point to the possibility of using small molecules to target mitochondrial dynamics in various circumstances to treat mitochondrial malfunction and the health issues that accompany it.

7.2 CRISPR-based Strategies for Modulation Future Perspectives.

Targeting the mitochondrial genome and modifying mitochondrial dynamics with CRISPR/Cas9 technology has demonstrated promise in bridging the gap between health and malfunction. Still, there are certain issues that need to be resolved. Among the salient features of the search results are:

Mitochondrial DNA has been edited using CRISPR/Cas9, which offers the potential to treat disorders related to the mitochondria.

A significant barrier is the dearth of efficient techniques for delivering guide RNA (gRNA), which is mostly dependent on tRNA, past the mitochondrial membrane.

The use of donated oocytes, preimplantation genetic diagnostics, and mitochondrial replacement therapy (MRT) are methods to stop the spread of mtDNA disorders.

The stringent PAM site requirement, off-target mutagenesis, and transport techniques into various cell types or animal models are challenges in applying CRISPR-based gene editing for mtDNA.

The CRISPR/Cas genome editing approach is limited to editing nuclear genomes and is not an effective way to alter mitochondrial genomes due to the lack of an efficient delivery route to import gRNA into the mitochondria.

In conclusion, even though CRISPR/Cas9 targets the mitochondrial genome with promise, more work needs to be done to fully realize its potential for modifying mitochondrial dynamics and treating disorders connected to the mitochondria. These challenges include the efficient delivery of gRNA into the mitochondria.

Chapter Eight

8.1 Emerging Research Avenues

Maintaining optimal mitochondrial function is largely dependent on mechanisms such as fission, fusion, mitophagy, and transport, which are all parts of mitochondrial dynamics. A variety of illnesses, such as cancer, metabolic, cardiovascular, and neurological disorders, are linked to imbalances in mitochondrial dynamics, which can result in aberrant cellular fate.

New studies in this area have found that mitofusin 2, dynamin-related protein 1, mitophagy, biogenesis, metformin, and inflammation are possible targets for therapeutic intervention. Research has also emphasized the significance of mitochondrial dynamics in neurodegeneration and neurogenetic illnesses, indicating that appropriate regulation of mitochondrial dynamics may offer a window for therapeutic intervention, especially in diseases like Alzheimer. In order to create more precise strategies for targeted regulation of mitochondrial activity, there is ongoing inquiry into the regulation of mitochondrial dynamics and its role in regulating cellular function.

8.2 Potential Implications for Disease Treatment Conclusion

Because they influence the structure of the mitochondrial network, aid in mitochondrial function, and maintain quality control, mitochondrial dynamics are important in bridging the gap between health and dysfunction.

Many illnesses, such as cardiac and neurodegenerative conditions, are linked to imbalanced mitochondrial dynamics. Function has been improved in a number of illness models by genetically or chemically altering mitochondrial fusion and division. Based on mitochondrial dynamics, the following possible therapy implications for diseases have been identified:

1. Slowing the progression of disease: Mitochondrial dynamics may promote health and slow the progression of disease by influencing essential mitochondrial functions.

2. Diminishing tissue deterioration and cellular dysfunction: Treatments that reinstate equilibrium in mitochondrial dynamics have the potential to mitigate morphological and functional irregularities as well as cellular dysfunction.

3. Personalized medicine: A deeper comprehension of the relationship between mitochondrial dynamics and changes in cellular state space may enable the development of a non-terminal imaging-based method for monitoring these changes, as well as help determine their nature

4. Comparing gene variants: It is possible to detect distinct and prevalent cellular phenotypes of disorders linked to mitochondrial dynamics by comparing the cellular effects of various gene variants related to mitochondrial dynamics in patients.

5. Aiming for targeted therapeutics for neurogenetic diseases: A growing knowledge of the malfunction of mitochondrial dynamics can aid in the development of targeted medicines for these conditions

6. Detailed plans for focused regulation: More accurate plans for focused regulation of mitochondrial function will be developed as a result of a thorough grasp of mitochondrial dynamics.

In conclusion, comprehending and adjusting mitochondrial dynamics presents auspicious therapeutic prospects for an extensive array of human ailments. Through focusing on mitochondrial fusion, division, and quality control, scientists may be able to decrease cellular malfunction, slow the advancement of disease, and enhance general health.

Chapter Nine

9.1 Summarizing the Key Findings

Fission, fusion, mitophagy, and transport are examples of the several aspects of mitochondrial dynamics that are critical to preserving optimal mitochondrial function, which is required for energy production and other critical cellular functions. The distribution of mitochondrial DNA, quality control, and metabolic status are all dependent on a balanced mitochondrial network. Any alteration to the dynamics of the mitochondria can result in aberrant cellular destiny and a variety of illnesses, such as cancer, metabolic, cardiovascular, and neurological diseases.

The identification of the machinery involved in mitochondrial dynamics and its malfunction in disease are important discoveries in the field of mitochondrial dynamics research. Parts of this apparatus include ocular atrophy protein 1 (OPA1), mitofusins 1 and 2 (MFN1, MFN2), and dynamin-related protein 1 (DRP1). Neurodegenerative illnesses can result from an imbalance in mitochondrial dynamics, and common diseases like type 2 diabetes are also associated with altered mitochondrial dynamics.

Understanding the molecular mechanisms governing mitochondrial dynamics is crucial for figuring out how mitochondrial shape meets function and for expanding our knowledge of the molecular underpinnings of diseases linked to morphology defects. Mitochondrial dynamics are critical for controlling decisions about the fate of cells.

In conclusion, mitochondrial dynamics are essential for bridging the gap between normalcy and pathology. Numerous diseases can result from imbalanced mitochondrial dynamics, yet it has been demonstrated that improving mitochondrial fitness through regulation of mitochondrial dynamics lowers the risk of disease and improves general health.

9.2 Looking Ahead: Implications for Cellular and Medical Research

The investigation of mitochondrial dynamics has uncovered a convoluted and interdependent system that is essential to preserving the best possible mitochondrial function. Unbalances in mitochondrial dynamics have been linked to a variety of illnesses, including neurodegenerative, neoplastic, endocrine, and cardiovascular diseases. Therefore, this has important implications for cellular and medical studies.

A more comprehensive approach to mitochondrial activity is necessary, and this is one of the main consequences for cellular and medical research. This entails taking into account the physiology of actual tissues in addition to creating experimental instruments that can adapt to the needs of researching living, breathing organelles like mitochondria.

Another implication is that in order to understand how mitochondrial form meets function and to learn more about the molecular basis of disorders linked to morphological abnormalities, it is imperative to comprehend the molecular mechanisms governing mitochondrial dynamics.

All things considered, research on mitochondrial dynamics has great promise for improving our knowledge of human health and illness as well as for generating fresh approaches to treating a variety of ailments.

Conclusion

In order to preserve cellular metabolic balance, cell death, and cell survival, mitochondrial dynamics are essential. They involve the molecular and mechanical processes of fission, fusion, and motility—all of which are necessary to preserve the homeostasis of the mitochondria. Numerous human diseases have been linked to dysfunction in mitochondrial dynamics, which makes mitochondria a viable pharmaceutical target for the therapy of a wide spectrum of diseases.

Important facets of the dynamics of mitochondria include:

Fusion and fission: These mechanisms regulate the size, quantity, and shape of mitochondria. The emergence of mitochondrial diseases can be significantly influenced by changes in mitochondrial dynamics.

Motility: The movement of mitochondria to locations with high energy requirements is facilitated by molecular and mechanical processes. In intracellular signaling, motility is also crucial.

Proteins involved: To sustain mitochondrial dynamics, proteins like OPA1, mitofusins 1 and 2, and dynamin-related protein 1 (DRP1) are essential. Depolarized mitochondria have been shown to have lower OPA1 levels in the intermembrane space.

Characterizing mitochondrial motility may be a valuable clinical indicator of dysfunctional mitochondrial dynamics that can be utilized to track the course of a disease or evaluate the efficacy of a treatment intervention. There is promise for better treatment of mitochondrial illnesses and related conditions thanks to developments in the understanding of mitochondrial dynamics and the creation of targeted medicines based on particular molecular factors.

Reference

Chan, D. C. (2012). Fusion and fission: Interlinked processes critical for mitochondrial health. Annual Review of Genetics, 46, 265-287.

Chen, H., & Chan, D. C. (2009). Mitochondrial dynamics—fusion, fission, movement, and mitophagy—in neurodegenerative diseases. Human Molecular Genetics, 18(R2), R169-R176.

Cogliati, S., Frezza, C., Soriano, M. E., Varanita, T., Quintana-Cabrera, R., Corrado, M., ... & Scorrano, L. (2013). Mitochondrial cristae shape determines respiratory chain supercomplexes assembly and respiratory efficiency. Cell, 155(1), 160-171.

Detmer, S. A., & Chan, D. C. (2007). Functions and dysfunctions of mitochondrial dynamics. Nature Reviews Molecular Cell Biology, 8(11), 870-879.

Liesa, M., & Shirihai, O. S. (2013). Mitochondrial dynamics in the regulation of nutrient utilization and energy expenditure. Cell Metabolism, 17(4), 491-506.

Mishra, P., & Chan, D. C. (2014). Metabolic regulation of mitochondrial dynamics. Journal of Cell Biology, 204(3), 391-399.

Nunnari, J., & Suomalainen, A. (2012). Mitochondria: In sickness and in health. Cell, 148(6), 1145-1159.

Twig, G., & Shirihai, O. S. (2011). The interplay between mitochondrial dynamics and mitophagy. Antioxidants & Redox Signaling, 14(10), 1939-1951.

Westermann, B. (2010). Mitochondrial fusion and fission in cell life and death. Nature Reviews Molecular Cell Biology, 11(12), 872-884.

Youle, R. J., & van der Bliek, A. M. (2012). Mitochondrial fission, fusion, and stress. Science, 337(6098), 1062-1065.

Yapa, N. M. B., & Lisnyak, T. (2021). Mitochondrial dynamics in health and disease. *FEBS Letters*, 595(8), 1113-1126. https://doi.org/10.1002/1873-3468.14077

Zhang, J., & Ney, P. A. (2023). Mitochondrial dynamics in health and disease: mechanisms and potential targets. *Cellular and Molecular Life Sciences*, 80(3), 337-348. https://doi.org/10.1007/s00018-021-04100-3